KLINEFELTER SYNDROME

THINGS YOU SHOULD KNOW

(QUESTIONS AND ANSWERS)

By Rumi Michael Leigh

Introduction

I would like to thank and congratulate you for purchasing this book, " *Klinefelter syndrome, things you should know (questions and answers)*" series.

This book will help you understand, revise and have a good general knowledge and keywords of Klinefelter syndrome.

Thanks again for purchasing this book, I hope you enjoy it!

Table of Contents

Section 1

1) What is Klinefelter syndrome?

- Klinefelter syndrome is the presence of an extra X chromosome in a male.

2) Is there a possibility to have more than one X chromosome in Klinefelter disease?

- Yes, there is a possibility to have more than one X chromosome in Klinefelter disease.

3) Is Klinefelter syndrome a genetic condition?

- Yes, Klinefelter syndrome is a genetic condition.

4) Is Klinefelter syndrome inherited?

- No, Klinefelter syndrome is not inherited.

5) Does Klinefelter syndrome affect females?

- No, Klinefelter syndrome does not affect females it affects only males.

6) Could a person have Klinefelter syndrome without knowing?

- Yes, a person could have Klinefelter syndrome without knowing.

7) Is there a cure for Klinefelter syndrome?

- No, there is no cure for Klinefelter syndrome.

8) Are there other names for Klinefelter syndrome?

- Yes, there are other names for Klinefelter syndrome.

9) What are other names for Klinefelter syndrome?

- Other names for Klinefelter syndrome include XXY syndrome, XXY trisomy, and 47.

10) Can people with Klinefelter syndrome lead a normal life?

- Yes, people with Klinefelter syndrome can lead a normal life.

Section 2

1) What is a chromosome?

- A chromosome is a long DNA molecule that contains the genetic material.

2) What is a gene?

- A gene is a segment of DNA.

3) How many pairs of chromosomes are there in the human body?

- There are 23 pairs of chromosomes in the human body.

4) What is the normal number of chromosomes in the human body?

- The normal number of chromosomes in the human body is 46.

5) What are autosomes?

- Autosomes are the 22 pairs of chromosomes in the 23 pairs of chromosomes in the human body.

6) What is the pair of the sex chromosomes?

- The sex chromosomes is the 23rd pair of chromosomes in the 23 pairs of chromosomes in the human body.

7) What are the sex chromosomes?

- The sex chromosomes are the X and Y chromosomes.

8) What are the chromosomes in a male?

- The chromosomes in a male are the XY chromosomes.

9) What are the chromosomes in a female?

- The chromosomes in a female are the XX chromosomes.

10) What are the chromosomes in a person with Klinefelter syndrome?

- A person with Klinefelter syndrome has XXY chromosomes.

Section 3

1) Can the extra X chromosome be carried in the sperm?

- Yes, the extra X chromosome can be carried in the sperm.

2) Can the extra X chromosome be carried in the egg?

- Yes, the extra X chromosome can be carried in the egg.

3) Is Klinefelter syndrome a common chromosomal sex disorder?

- Yes, Klinefelter syndrome is a common chromosomal sex disorder.

4) Are the symptoms of Klinefelter syndrome always the same?

- No, the symptoms of Klinefelter syndrome are not always the same, symptoms may vary.

5) What are the signs and symptoms of Klinefelter syndrome?

- The signs and symptoms of Klinefelter syndrome are weak bones and muscles, low energy, very low sperm count, small testicles, absent puberty, delayed puberty or incomplete puberty, delayed speech, less facial hair, less body hair, dyslexia, infertility, long legs, feminine hip structure, difficulty in social interactions, etc.

6) What is hypogonadism?

- Hypogonadism is the decreased production of testosterone.

7) What is dyslexia?

- Dyslexia is a learning difficulty. Difficulties such as reading, writing, spelling, and speaking.

8) What is dyspraxia?

- Dyspraxia is a neurological disorder that affects motor skills.

9) What is the most common symptom of Klinefelter syndrome?

- The most common symptom of Klinefelter syndrome is infertility.

10) Do the signs and symptoms of Klinefelter syndrome also depend on the person's age?

- Yes, the signs and symptoms of Klinefelter syndrome also depend on the person's age.

Section 4

1) When are the symptoms of Klinefelter syndrome usually noticed?

- The symptoms of Klinefelter syndrome are usually noticed during puberty.

2) What can worsen the symptoms of Klinefelter syndrome?

- The presence of more X chromosomes can worsen symptoms of Klinefelter syndrome.

3) What is aneuploidy?

- Aneuploidy is an abnormal number of chromosomes in a cell.

4) What is gynecomastia?

- Gynecomastia is the enlarged breasts in men.

5) What is osteoporosis?

- Osteoporosis is a disease that causes loss in bone density.

6) What is a major complication for osteoporosis?

- Osteoporosis can lead to bone fracture.

7) What is a congenital disease?

- A congenital disease is a disease that a person is born with.

8) Can Klinefelter syndrome lead to anxiety?

- Yes, Klinefelter syndrome can lead to anxiety.

9) Can Klinefelter syndrome lead to depression?

- Yes, Klinefelter syndrome can lead to depression.

Section 5

1) Can Klinefelter syndrome lead to diabetes mellitus?

- Yes, Klinefelter syndrome can lead to diabetes mellitus.

2) What is diabetes mellitus?

- Diabetes mellitus is a disease that causes abnormally high blood glucose levels.

3) Diabetes mellitus is also called?

- Diabetes mellitus is also called diabetes.

4) Can Klinefelter syndrome lead to varicose veins?

- Yes, Klinefelter syndrome can lead to varicose veins.

5) What are varicose veins?

- Varicose veins are enlarged and twisted veins.

6) Can varicose veins be found everywhere in the body?

- Yes, varicose veins can be found everywhere in the body.

7) Can Klinefelter syndrome lead to hypothyroidism?

- Yes, Klinefelter syndrome can lead to hypothyroidism.

8) What is hypothyroidism?

- Hypothyroidism is an insufficiency of the production of thyroid hormones.

9) Could Klinefelter syndrome increase the risk of breast cancer?

- Yes, Klinefelter syndrome could increase the risk of breast cancer.

10) Could Klinefelter syndrome lead to ophthalmic issues?

- Yes, Klinefelter syndrome could lead to ophthalmic issues.

11) Could Klinefelter syndrome lead to cardiac issues?

- Yes, Klinefelter syndrome could lead to cardiac issues.

Section 6

1) What is testosterone?

- Testosterone is the male sex hormone.

2) What is cryptorchidism?

- Cryptorchidism is a small testes or undescendent testes.

3) Testes are also called?

- Testes are also called testicles.

4) What is hypospadias?

- Hypospadias is a malformation of the opening of the penis.

5) What is azoospermia?

- Azoospermia is the absence of sperm in the semen.

6) What is oligospermia?

- Oligospermia is a low sperm count.

7) What is oogenesis?

- Oogenesis is the creation of the female gamete.

8) Oogenesis is also known as?

- Oogenesis is also known as ovogenesis.

9) What is spermatogenesis?

- Spermatogenesis is the creation of the male gamete.

10) What is lethargy?

- Lethargy is severe fatigue and low energy.

Section 7

1) What are the ova?

- The ova are the female gamete.

2) What is the male gamete?

- The male gamete is the sperm.

3) Do males and females have gonads?

- Yes, males and females have gonads.

4) What are the male gonads?

- The male gonads are the testicles.

5) What are the female gonads?

- The female gonads are the ovaries.

6) Can Klinefelter syndrome be diagnosed before birth?

- Yes, Klinefelter syndrome can be diagnosed before birth.

7) How can Klinefelter syndrome be diagnosed before birth?

- Klinefelter syndrome can be diagnosed before birth by testing the mother.

8) What is amniocentesis?

- Amniocentesis is a medical procedure for test purposes that involves extracting a sample of amniotic fluid.

9) What is the main function of the amniotic fluid?

- The main function of the amniotic fluid is the protection of the fetus.

10) What is chorionic villus sampling?

- Chorionic villus sampling is a medical test done during pregnancy where a sample of chorionic villi is taken from the placenta in order to check for abnormalities in the body.

Section 8

1) How is Klinefelter syndrome diagnosed?

- Klinefelter syndrome is diagnosed by blood test for chromosome analysis, infertility test in men.

2) What is karyotype?

- Karyotype is the analysis of chromosomes.

3) Can Klinefelter syndrome lead to auto-immune disorders?

- Yes, Klinefelter syndrome can lead to auto-immune disorders.

4) What is an autoimmune disease?

- An autoimmune disease is when the immune system of the body attacks the body.

5) What are some examples of autoimmune diseases?

- Some examples of autoimmune diseases are lupus, rheumatoid arthritis, Sjogren's syndrome, etc.

6) What is lupus?

- Lupus is an autoimmune disease that causes inflammation in the body.

7) Lupus is also called?

- Lupus is also called systemic lupus erythematosus.

8) What is rheumatoid arthritis?

- Rheumatoid arthritis is a chronic inflammation of the joints.

9) What is Sjogren syndrome?

- Sjogren syndrome is an autoimmune disease that causes dry eyes and dry mouth.

Section 9

1) What are some variants of Klinefelter syndrome?

- Some variants of Klinefelter syndrome are 48, XXXY, 49XXXXY, etc.

2) What is mosaic Klinefelter syndrome?

- Mosaic Klinefelter syndrome is the presence of an extra X chromosome in some cells.

3) What is the most common Klinefelter syndrome karyotype?

- The most common Klinefelter syndrome karyotype is 47XXY.

4) Can Klinefelter syndrome be treated?

- Yes, Klinefelter syndrome can be treated.

5) What are the treatments for Klinefelter syndrome?

- The treatments for Klinefelter syndrome include fertility treatment, testosterone replacement therapy, speech and language therapy, physical therapy, occupational therapy, etc.

6) What is nondisjunction?

- Nondisjunction is the failure of correct chromosomes separation.

7) What is meiosis?

- Meiosis is cell division.

Section 10

1) What is estradiol?

- Estradiol is an estrogen hormone.

2) Estradiol could also be called?

- Estradiol could also be called oestradiol.

3) Is estradiol a steroid hormone?

- Yes, estradiol is a steroid hormone.

4) How are estradiol levels in a person with Klinefelter syndrome?

- Estradiol levels are high in a person with Klinefelter syndrome.

5) How are testosterone levels in a person with Klinefelter syndrome?

- Testosterone levels are low in a person with Klinefelter syndrome.

6) What is the luteinizing hormone?

- Luteinizing hormone is a hormone involved in puberty and the menstrual cycle.

7) What is the level of luteinizing hormone in a person with Klinefelter syndrome?

- In a person with Klinefelter syndrome, luteinizing hormone is high.

8) Where is the luteinizing hormone produced?

- Luteinizing hormone is a glycoprotein hormone that is produced in the anterior pituitary gland.

9) Where is the pituitary gland located?

- The pituitary gland is located in the brain.

10) The pituitary gland can also be called?

- The pituitary gland can also be called hypophysis.

11) What is the follicle-stimulating hormone?

- The follicle-stimulating hormones are gonadotropins produced by the pituitary gland. Follicle-stimulating hormones aid in reproduction.

12) What is the level of follicle-stimulating hormone in a person with Klinefelter syndrome?

- In a person with Klinefelter syndrome, the follicle-stimulating hormone is high.

Conclusion

Thank you again for purchasing this book. I hope it has helped you in your journey to understanding Klinefelter syndrome and its effects on the body.

Please, if you enjoyed this book, I would like you to rate and comment. It'd be appreciated.

Thank you.